THE DOCTOR'S OATH

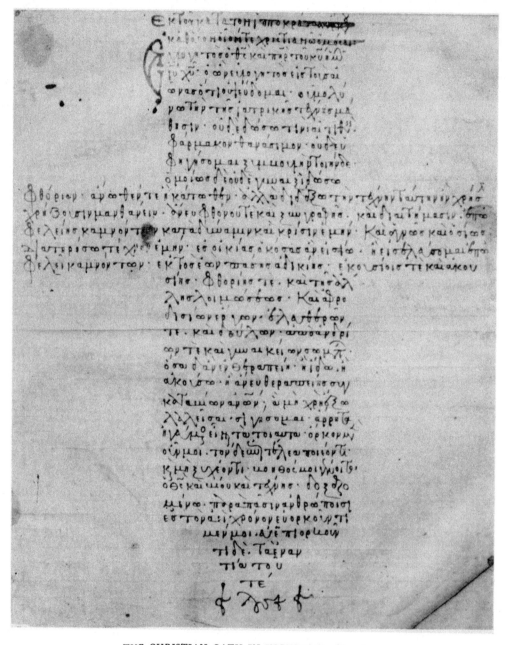

THE CHRISTIAN OATH IN URBINAS 64, *fol.* 116

THE DOCTOR'S OATH

AN ESSAY IN THE HISTORY OF MEDICINE

By

W. H. S. JONES, M.A.

BURSAR OF S. CATHARINE'S COLLEGE,
CAMBRIDGE, CORRESPONDING MEMBER
OF THE ROYAL SOCIETY OF
MEDICINE

CAMBRIDGE
AT THE UNIVERSITY PRESS
MCMXXIV

ὠφελεῖν ἢ μὴ βλάπτειν.

HIPPOCRATES *Epid.* i. v

CONTENTS

CAMBRIDGE
UNIVERSITY PRESS

University Printing House, Cambridge CB2 8BS, United Kingdom

Published in the United States of America by Cambridge University Press, New York

Cambridge University Press is part of the University of Cambridge.

It furthers the University's mission by disseminating knowledge in the pursuit of
education, learning and research at the highest international levels of excellence.

www.cambridge.org
Information on this title: www.cambridge.org/9781107627307

© Cambridge University Press 1924

First published 1924
First paperback edition 2013

A catalogue record for this publication is available from the British Library

ISBN 978-1-107-62730-7 Paperback

PREFACE

I HAVE written this little book for physicians and surgeons, that they may have the earliest forms of that famous oath upon which the ethical rules of their profession have been based. Perhaps, too, the documents that I have collected will be of some interest to scholars and to historians of medicine. I have at least shown that an enormous amount of "spade work" remains to be done for the Hippocratic Collection.

I believe that Marcianus Venetus 269 is the only important manuscript of *Oath* cited in critical editions. The others usually cited are all unimportant Paris manuscripts. The Christian oath has never been published before.

The task of collating over thirty manuscripts has not been easy, and I wish to thank many officials in the great libraries of Europe, in particular the Librarian of the Ambrosian Library at Milan and Professor Rostagno of Florence, for their kindness and courtesy. Many Cambridge friends have helped me in my efforts to throw light upon dark places, and I am under a special obligation to Dr E. T. Withington of Oxford, who for fourteen years has been generous to a degree in helping me in my study of Greek medicine.

The design on the cover is from a mediaeval portrait of Hippocrates in the Bologna manuscript Bononiensis 3632.

W. H. S. J.

May 1924

THE MANUSCRIPTS OF THE
HIPPOCRATIC COLLECTION

THE MANUSCRIPTS OF THE HIPPOCRATIC COLLECTION

THE Hippocratic Collection is a miscellany of books which probably represents the library of the Coan school of medicine. Losses on the one hand, and additions on the other, have resulted in the extant *corpus*, which contains some seventy works[1].

Many of these books were for centuries the practical manuals of medical students and doctors, and it is not surprising that the manuscripts are many and various[2]. None of them, however, contains the whole *corpus*, though the two Paris manuscripts, 2255 and 2254, written by the same scribe in the fifteenth century, omit when taken together very little that is included in Littré's nine volumes. Some manuscripts contain thirty or more treatises, some several, others only one.

The manuscripts may be divided roughly into three classes.

(1) Our best authorities:

    (*a*) Vindobonensis med. IV (θ) xth cent.
    (*b*) Parisinus 2253 (A) xith cent.
    (*c*) Parisinus 446 suppl. (C′) xth cent.
    (*d*) Laurentianus 74, 7 (B) xth cent. (?)[3].

---

[1] Jones *Hippocrates* I pp. xxii–xxx.
[2] *Ibid.* p. lxiii.
[3] None of these manuscripts contains *Oath*.

As no treatise is common to any two of these manuscripts, it is impossible to decide whether they represent one "family" or more than one. Perhaps Urbinas 64 ought to be included in this class, but as far as I can judge the text it gives is not quite so pure as that of the other four[1].

(2) Vaticanus Graecus 276[2], and the manuscripts closely allied to it, if not actually copied from it, namely Parisinus 2146, Holkhamensis 282 and Palatino-Vaticanus 192[3].

(3) Marcianus Venetus 269[4], and the manuscripts allied to it, which include most of the *recentiores*, more or less "edited."

A study of the Hippocratic text will convince any inquirer that it has not been preserved with verbal fidelity. At some period, or periods, in the history of the text, little care seems to have been given to literal faithfulness provided that the general sense was kept. There was no spirit of reverence among the possessors of manuscripts like that which has kept comparatively pure the text of many classical authors. The Hippocratic works are text-books, not literary master-

---

[1] It appears to me to be very closely allied to Littré's "S," an early Paris MS (Paris. 2228). I base this conclusion on my collation of *Aphorisms* in Urb. 64. The Milan manuscript Ambros. B 113 sup. contains much the same collection of works, including an excerpt from Περὶ φυσῶν.

[2] See below, p. 4.

[3] Holk. 282 and Paris. 2146 were written by the same scribe. The handwritings are without doubt identical. Dr Minns after a close examination confirms my view.

[4] See p. 4.

pieces. Hence transpositions of words, glosses, interpolations, are more than usually common. Is there any parallel to the freedom with which the writer of the Christian oath treated his original?

MANUSCRIPTS OF OATH

The best manuscripts containing *Oath* are the following:

(1) Urbinas 64 fol. 116 (in the Vatican Library), a manuscript of the tenth or eleventh century. It is very different from the manuscripts which follow, as it contains *Oath* modified "so that a Christian may take it." Its version of *Oath* is given in facsimile as frontispiece.

(2) Marcianus Venetus 269 (M) fol. 12, an eleventh-century manuscript in the Library of St Mark at Venice.

(3) Vaticanus Graecus 276 (V) fol. 1, a twelfth-century manuscript in the Vatican Library at Rome.

I have collated these manuscripts from rotographs.

The later manuscripts are:

(1) The Christian form:

> Ambros. B 113 sup. (xivth cent.) fol. 203v. A facsimile is given on p. 26.
> Bonon. 3632 (xvth cent.) fol. 28.

(2) The usual form:

> Paris MSS: 2140 (xiith–xiiith cent.)[1] fol. 9v.
> 2142 (xiiith–xivth cent.)[2] fol. 12v.

---

[1] So Diels. Littré (I 521) puts the date a century later.

[2] The part containing *Oath* is in the later of the two hands in which this MS is written.

2143 (xivth cent.) fol. 11.
2144 (xivth cent.) fol. 13.
2596 (xivth cent.) fol. 185ᵛ
2047 (xvth cent.) fol. 16.
2141 (xvth cent.) fol. 8ᵛ.
2145 (xvth cent.) fol. 14.
2148 (xvth cent.) fol. 1.
2255 (xvth cent.) fol. 55.
2146 (xvith cent.) fol. 1.
Suppl. gr. 608 (xvith cent.) fol. 178ᵛ.

Rome MSS: Urbinas 68 (xivth cent.) fol. 16.
Vaticanus 277 (xivth cent.) fol. 25.
Palatinus 192 (xvth cent.) fol. 1.
Reg. Suec. 182 (xvth cent.) fol. 16.
Vaticanus 2238 (xvth cent.) fol. 180.

Florence MSS: Laurentianus plut. 74, 1 (xvth cent.)
fol. 9ᵛ.
Laurentianus plut. 74, 13 (xvth cent.)
fol. 7.

Milan MS: Ambrosianus B 113 sup.[1] (xivth cent.) fol. 2.

London MSS: Arundel 538 (xvth cent.) fol. 19.
Stowe 1073 (xvith cent.) fol. 2.

Oxford MSS: Baroccian 204 (xvth cent.) fol. 9.
Miscell. 132 (xvith cent.) fol. 1.

Vienna MS: Vindobonensis 4772 fol. 105.

Prague MS: Vindobonensis Philol. 219 (xivth cent.) fol. 140.

Escurial MS: Scorialensis Σ II 5 (xvth cent.) fol. 28ᵛ.

Cambridge MS: Caius 50 (xvth–xvith cent.) fol. 1.

There are also sixteenth-century MSS at Athos (ΒΙΒΛ. ΜΟΝ.

---

[1] There is in the Escurial a copy of this manuscript made in the sixteenth century, when the original was not in Milan but in Venice. See Dietz *Scholia in Hippocratem et Galenum* II pp. v and vi.

IBHP. 4302.182 fol. 8ᵛ), Leyden (Voss. fol. 10), and at Copenhagen (Hauniens. ant. fund. reg. 224).

Nearly all the *recentiores* appear to be closely related to M or V, mostly the former.

The descriptions of the manuscripts I have taken from Diels[1]. His foliation is often wrong[2], and where possible I have corrected it.

For the pagan oath I have recorded the readings of M, V and R (Vaticanus Graecus 277), a fourteenth-century manuscript which is perhaps the best of the *recentiores*.

In making my *apparatus criticus* I have noticed every variant, with the exception of punctuation marks, accents and omitted iota subscript.

Neither M nor V has any notes, but R has several. There is a long marginal note on γενέτῃσιν, which Littré quotes from the margin of Paris. 2255 (E). It has μάρτυρας written over ἵστορας, συμφωνίαν over ξυγγραφήν, συμφωνίας over ξυγγραφῆς and some case of παράκλησις over παραγγελίης. In the margin ὑποθήσομαι συμβουλίην is written as an explanation of ὑφηγήσομαι ξυμβουλίην.

---

[1] *Die Handschriften der antiken Ärzte.*

[2] E.g. "Laurent. plut. 74, 3 p. 188 b" should be "fol. 191ᵛ," and the version is that given on p. 57. So too Vat. 2304 [once 2217] fol. 1 contains the same metrical oath, with an extra line after ὀπάζειν, which seems to be:

οὔτε χάριν φιλίης ἑτέρῳ κακὰ νεῖμαι ὑπο....

Diels, however, gives it as a manuscript of the ordinary oath. The Librarian of the Estense Library, Modena, has sent me a transcript of Mutinensis 61 fol. 29ᵛ. It too contains the metrical oath. Again, *Oath* is on fol. 16 of Urbinas 68, not on fol. 4, as Diels says. Vindobonensis Philol. 219 is at Prague, not Vienna. This list of errors shows how much spade work remains to be done for the Hippocratic Collection.

The text printed below does not pretend to be more than an attempt to reproduce the archetype of M, V and R—in other words the *textus receptus* of mediaeval times. In two respects at least the printed text must be faulty:

(1) The aorists ἡγήσασθαι, κοινώσασθαι, ποιήσασθαι cannot be co-ordinate with the futures ἐπικρινεῖν and διδάξειν.

(2) The infinitive εἴρξειν cannot be co-ordinate with the indicative χρήσομαι.

I have, however, left these errors in the text because, although it would be easy enough to write something grammatical with the required sense, yet they appear to represent a combination or conflation of earlier forms, and it is not yet possible, if it ever will be possible, to determine what these forms originally were. Fortunately the uncertainty of the text does not represent a corresponding uncertainty of the sense.

The spelling has been modified so as to follow the rules laid down in the Teubner edition of Hippocrates (Kühlewein).

ΙΠΠΟΚΡΑΤΟΥС ΟΡΚΟС

Ὀμνύω Ἀπόλλωνα ἰητρὸν καὶ Ἀσκληπιὸν καὶ Ὑγείαν καὶ
Πανάκειαν καὶ θεοὺς πάντας τε καὶ πάσας, ἵστορας ποιεύμενος,
ἐπιτελέα ποιήσειν κατὰ δύναμιν καὶ κρίσιν ἐμὴν ὅρκον τόνδε καὶ
συγγραφὴν τήνδε·
5 †ἡγήσασθαί τε τὸν διδάξαντά με τὴν τέχνην ταύτην ἴσα γενέτῃσιν
ἐμοῖσι, καὶ βίου κοινώσασθαι, καὶ χρεῶν χρηΐζοντι μετάδοσιν
ποιήσασθαι, καὶ γένος τὸ ἐξ αὐτοῦ ἀδελφοῖς ἴσον ἐπικρινεῖν ἄρρεσι,
καὶ διδάξειν τὴν τέχνην ταύτην, ἢν χρηΐζωσι μανθάνειν, ἄνευ
μισθοῦ καὶ συγγραφῆς, παραγγελίης τε καὶ ἀκροήσιος καὶ τῆς
10 λοιπῆς ἁπάσης μαθήσιος μετάδοσιν ποιήσασθαι †υἱοῖσί τε ἐμοῖσι
καὶ τοῖσι τοῦ ἐμὲ διδάξαντος, καὶ μαθητῇσι συγγεγραμμένοις τε
καὶ ὡρκισμένοις νόμῳ ἰητρικῷ, ἄλλῳ δὲ οὐδενί.
διαιτήμασί τε χρήσομαι ἐπ' ὠφελείῃ καμνόντων κατὰ δύναμιν
καὶ κρίσιν ἐμήν, ἐπὶ δηλήσει δὲ καὶ ἀδικίῃ †εἴρξειν†.

---

1. 1 ὀμνύω MV ὄμνυμι R. 2 πάντας τε MR ἅπαντας V. 2, 3 So MR.
V has ἵστορας· ποιεύμενος ἐπιτελέα ποίησιν. 4 συγγραφὴν V (with ξ written
over the σ) ξυγγραφὴν MR. 5 τε V δὲ MR. R adds καὶ after ἴσα and
reads γενέταισιν. Probably the aorists ἡγήσασθαι, κοινώσασθαι, ποιήσασθαι
should be changed to futures. 6 ἐμοῖσι VR ἐμοῖσιν M. χρεῶν MR χρέους V,
which also reads χρήζοντι. 7 ἑωϋτέου MR. V omits καὶ γένος το μετάδοσιν
ποιήσασθαι. ἐπικρινέειν MR. 9 ξυγγραφῆς M ξυγγραφῆς R. 11 μαθηταῖσι MVR. 12 M has ὡρκιζσμένοις, the three dots meaning that -ζ- is
to be considered erased. 14 ἐπὶ δηλήσει VR ἐπιδηλήσει M. εἴρξειν MV
εἴρξειν R. Perhaps εἴρξω should be read.

PAGAN OATH

TRANSLATION

I swear by Apollo Physician, by Asclepius, by Health, by Heal-all, and by all the gods and goddesses, making them witnesses, that I will carry out, according to my ability and judgment, this oath and this indenture:

To regard my teacher in this art as equal to my parents; to make him partner in my livelihood, and when he is in need of money to share mine with him; to consider his offspring equal to my brothers; to teach them this art, if they require to learn it, without fee or indenture[1]; and to impart precept, oral instruction, and all the other learning[2], to my sons, to the sons of my teacher, and to pupils who have signed the indenture and sworn obedience to the physicians' Law, but to none other.

I will use treatment to help the sick according to my ability and judgment, but I will never use it[3] to injure or wrong them.

---

[1] It is uncertain whether the συγγραφὴ is a part of our extant text. It is the same as the indenture mentioned a little later on, and possibly refers to the deed of apprenticeship between master and pupil, and not to *Oath*.

[2] These strange phrases probably mean:

   (a) παραγγελίη, general rules of the art of medicine, as given for instance in *Precepts* (Παραγγελίαι).

   (b) ἀκρόησις, oral instruction, probably esoteric.

   (c) ἡ λοιπὴ μάθησις, practical instruction given in the surgery, like our "walking the hospitals."

[3] The construction probably is, "I will keep away all treatment which is intended to cause injury or wrong."

15 οὐ δώσω δὲ οὐδὲ φάρμακον οὐδενὶ αἰτηθεὶς θανάσιμον, οὐδὲ
ὑφηγήσομαι συμβουλίην τοιήνδε· ὁμοίως δὲ οὐδὲ γυναικὶ πεσσὸν
φθόριον δώσω· ἁγνῶς δὲ καὶ ὁσίως διατηρήσω βίον ἐμὸν καὶ
τέχνην ἐμήν.

οὐ τεμέω δὲ οὐδὲ μὴν λιθιῶντας, ἐκχωρήσω δὲ ἐργάτῃσιν ἀνδράσι
20 πρήξιος τῆσδε.

ἐς οἰκίας δὲ ὁκόσας ἂν ἐσίω, ἐσελεύσομαι ἐπ' ὠφελείῃ καμνόντων,
ἐκτὸς ἐὼν πάσης ἀδικίης ἑκουσίης καὶ φθορίης, τῆς τε ἄλλης καὶ
ἀφροδισίων ἔργων ἐπί τε γυναικείων σωμάτων καὶ ἀνδρείων,
ἐλευθέρων τε καὶ δούλων.

25 ἃ δ' ἂν ἐν θεραπείῃ ἢ ἴδω ἢ ἀκούσω, ἢ καὶ ἄνευ θεραπείης κατὰ
βίον ἀνθρώπων, ἃ μὴ χρή ποτε ἐκλαλεῖσθαι ἔξω, σιγήσομαι, ἄρρητα
ἡγεύμενος εἶναι τὰ τοιαῦτα.

ὅρκον μὲν οὖν μοι τόνδε ἐπιτελέα ποιέοντι, καὶ μὴ συγχέοντι,
εἴη ἐπαύρασθαι καὶ βίου καὶ τέχνης δοξαζομένῳ παρὰ πᾶσιν
30 ἀνθρώποις ἐς τὸν ἀεὶ χρόνον, παραβαίνοντι δὲ καὶ ἐπιορκέοντι
τἀναντία τούτων.

l. 16 ξυμβουλίην MVR. 16, 17 So MV. φθόριον δώσω πεσσόν R. 17, 18 So
MV. R places τὸν before ἐμὸν and τὴν before ἐμήν. 19 ἀνδράσι VR ἀνδράσιν M.
In V (as usual) πρήξιος appears as πρήξιος. 21 ἐς V εἰς MR. 23 ἀνδρείων MV
ἀνδρώων R. 25 V omits ἢ before ἴδω: perhaps rightly. M and R have
θεραπηίης. 26 ἐκλαλέεσθαι MVR. 27 εἶναι τὰ τοιαῦτα MR τὰ τοιαῦτα
εἶναι V. 28 ξυγχέοντι MVR. 30 ἐς V εἰς MR. ἀεὶ V αἰεὶ MR. ἐπιορκοῦντι MVR. 31 τουτέων MVR.

I will not give poison to anyone though asked to do so, nor will I suggest such a plan. Similarly I will not give a pessary to a woman to cause abortion. But in purity and in holiness I will guard my life and my art.

I will not use the knife either[1] on sufferers from stone, but I will give place to such as are craftsmen therein.

Into whatsoever houses I enter, I will do so to help the sick, keeping myself free from all intentional wrong-doing and harm, especially from fornication with woman or man, bond or free.

Whatsoever in the course of practice I see or hear (or even outside my practice in social intercourse) that ought never to be published abroad, I will not divulge, but consider such things to be holy secrets.

Now if I keep this oath and break it not, may I enjoy honour, in my life and art, among all men for all time; but if I transgress and forswear myself, may the opposite befall me.

[1] Perhaps, "I will not use the knife even on sufferers from stone."

THE LATER MANUSCRIPTS

It will be convenient to notice here the chief variants in the later manuscripts that I have either collated myself or had collated for me[1].

I may note that all have the aorists ἡγήσασθαι etc., μαθηταῖσι and ἐπιορκοῦντι.

BAROCCIAN 204. l. 1 ὄμνυμι. l. 5 ἡγήσασθαι δὲ: γονέησιν. l. 7 αυτέου. ἀδελφέοις. l. 14 ἀδικᾶν or ἀδικεῖν. l. 23 ἀνδρείων. l. 26 ἐκλέξασθαι.
The collation of this manuscript and of Miscell. 132 was made by Dr Withington.

MISCELL. 132 BODLEIAN. l. 1 ὀμνύω. l. 2 θεούς θ' ἅπαντας. l. 5 ἡγήσασθαί τε μεν. l. 6 χρέους χρηΐζοντι. Omits all between first μετάδοσιν ποιήσασθαι and second. l. 16 τήνδε. l. 17 τηρήσω. l. 23 ἀνδρείων. l. 25 ἢ ἄνευ. l. 27 τὰ τοιαῦτα εἶναι. This manuscript obviously belongs to the V class, but, unlike Paris. 2146 and Holkhamensis, it appears to have been "edited," as it contains several readings differing from those in V.

CAIUS 50. l. 1 ὄμνυμι. l. 5 μὲν. l. 6 μεταδίδωσιν. l. 12 ἄλλο δὲ οὐδενί. l. 16 ξυμβουλίαν. l. 23 ἀνδρείων.

ARUNDEL 538. l. 1 ὄμνυμι: ὑγείην. l. 5 δὲ: ἴσα καὶ. l. 7 ἑωϋτέου (pseudo-ionic?). l. 14 ἐπιδηλήσει. l. 15 οὐ δώσω δὲ οὐδενί. ll. 17, 18 τὸν ἐμὸν and τὴν ἐμήν. l. 20 πρήξιος. l. 21 εἰς.

STOWE 1073. l. 1 ὀμνύω. l. 2 θεοὺς θ' ἅπαντας καὶ. l. 5 τε. ll. 6–10 omits καὶ βίου to ἐμοῖσι—the scribe had the text of V in front of him, and his eye passed from γενέτῃσιν ἐμοῖσι to υἱοῖσί τε ἐμοῖσι. The omitted words are written in another hand in the margin,

---

[1] The readings of the Paris manuscripts can be found in Littré and Pétrequin.

but χρεων (sic) has ους written over -ων. This is an interesting combination of the M tradition and the V tradition. l. 16 τήνδε altered to τοιήνδε. l. 17 τηρήσω[1], as in Miscell. 132 Bodleian. ll. 17, 18 βίον τὸν ἐμὸν καὶ τέχνην ἐμήν. l. 20 πρήξηος with ϊ over -η-. l. 21 ἐσελεύσωμαι, a reading which seems to show that the ἢ before ἐσελεύσομαι in the Christian oath arose from the idea that ἐσελεύσομαι was a gloss on ἐσίω. l. 25 ἢ before ἴδω omitted. καὶ is omitted but is added in the margin. l. 27 τὰ τοιαῦτα εἶναι. This is a most interesting manuscript, obviously of the V class, and very closely related to Miscell. 132 Bodleian. All the late manuscripts of this class that I have seen (Paris. 2146, Holkhamensis 282, Miscell. 132, Stowe 1073) are of the fifteenth or sixteenth century. Apparently this family became popular about the year 1500 A.D. instead of the M family, which gave us our *textus receptus* of most of the Hippocratic Collection. I think this MS reads ξυμβουλὴν (l. 16).

PARIS. 2146. l. 1 ὀμνύω. l. 3 ποίησιν altered to ποιήσειν. l. 7 καὶ γένος.... l. 10 ποιήσασθαι omitted. l. 10 (after ἐμοῖσι) καὶ βίου κοινώσασθαι with erasure-dots under the last two words. l. 12 ἄλλῳ οὐδενί. l. 16 πεσὸν φθόριον δώσω. l. 19 ἀνδράσιν. l. 20 πρήξηος. l. 25 ἢ omitted before ἴδω. l. 27 τὰ τοιαῦτα εἶναι. l. 28 μοι omitted. This manuscript was probably copied from V.

PARIS. 2140. l. 1 ὄμνυμι. l. 5 δὲ : ἴσα. l. 7 ἐωῦτέου (apparently) like Arundel 538. l. 14 ἐπιδηλήσει. ll. 17, 18 βίον τὸν ἐμὸν καὶ τέχνην τὴν ἐμήν. l. 21 εἰς. l. 23 ἀνδρείων. l. 30 εἰς. This is a manuscript very typical of the later manuscript tradition, though it is perhaps as early as 1300 A.D. It is unlike V, and combines the peculiarities of M and R, with a leaning towards R.

PARIS. SUPPL. GR. 608 (not collated by Littré). l. 1 ὄμνυμι: ὑγείην. l. 3 ἐπιτελὲς: ἐμόν. l. 5 δὲ: ἴσα καὶ. l. 7 ἐωντέου: ἴσον. l. 8 ἢν χρηΐωσι ἄνευ. l. 11 καὶ τοῦ ἐμὲ. l. 14 ἐπιδήλησι δὲ καὶ ἀδικίῳ.

---

[1] διατηρήσω in margin. Just above, ξυγγραφῆς is glossed by ξυμφωνίας, and παραγγελίης by παρακλήσεως. Cf. the glosses in R, p. 6.

l. 15 οὐ δώσω δὲ οὐδενὶ φάρμακον αἰτθεὶς τανάσιμον. l. 17 τὸν ἐμὸν. l. 18 τὴν ἐμὴν. l. 21 εἰς: ὠφιλείη. l. 30 εἰς: αἰεὶ. This is a manuscript similar to Paris. 2140 and also to Arundel 538.

LAURENTIANUS PLUT. 74, 1. l. 1 ὄμνυμι. l. 5 ἡγήσασθαι δὲ. l. 7 ἴσον. l. 14 ἐπιδηλήσει. l. 17 τὸν ἐμὸν. l. 18 τὴν ἐμὴν. This is a typical *recentior*—a mixture of M and R.

LAURENTIANUS PLUT. 74, 13. l. 1 ὄμνυμι. l. 5 ἡγήσασθαι μὲν, τὸν. l. 5 ἴσα καὶ γενέτοισιν. l. 7 ὠυτέου: ἀποκρινέειν. l. 16 ὁμοίως οὐδὲ. ll. 16, 17 γυναικὶ φθόριον δώσω πεσσόν. l. 26 ἐκκαλέεσθαι. l. 27 ἡγούμενος. l. 28 omits καὶ μὴ συγχέοντι. This is a MS akin to R.

The collation of 74, 1 and of 74, 13 was communicated by Professor Rostagno.

URBINAS 68. l. 1 ὄμνυμι. l. 5 δὲ: ἴσα καὶ γενέτοισιν ἐμοῖσι. l. 7 ὠυτέου. l. 14 ἐπιδηλήσει with βλάβη as gloss *supra*. l. 16 φθόριον δώσω πεσσὸν. l. 17 τὸν ἐμὸν. l. 18 τὴν ἐμὴν. l. 23 ἀνδρώων. l. 26 ἐκκαλέεσθαι. l. 30 εἰς: αἰεὶ. There are several marginal and interlinear notes similar to those in Vaticanus Gr. 277 (R). The close resemblance of the two manuscripts makes me doubt whether I read R aright in l. 5. I have given γενέταισιν in the *apparatus criticus*, but it might be γενέτοισιν, and that is certainly the reading of Urbinas 68.

REG. SUEC. 182. l. 1 ὄμνυμι. l. 5 δὲ: ἴσα καὶ γενέτησιν ἐμοῖσι. l. 7 ἑωυτέου: ἴσον. l. 9 παραγγελίης is written in a cramped way, so that it might easily be misread as παιγνίης. So apparently it was read by one of the Latin translators. See p. 37. l. 17 τὸν ἐμὸν. l. 18 τὴν ἐμὴν. l. 30 εἰς: αἰεὶ.

VATICANUS GRAECUS 2238. l. 1 ὄμνυμι. l. 5 δὲ: ἴσα γενέτησιν. l. 7 ἑωιτοῦ: ἴσον. l. 12 ὠρκισμένοις. l. 17 ἀγνῶς: τὸν ἐμὸν. l. 18 τὴν ἐμὴν. l. 19 ἀνδράσι. l. 30 εἰς: αἰεὶ.

VINDOBONENSIS 4772. l. 1 ὄμνυμι. l. 5 ἴσα καὶ. l. 26 ἐκκαλέεσθαι. Smooth breathing for rough breathing in many places. The collation of this manuscript was sent by Dr Karl Mras.

Vɪɴᴅᴏʙᴏɴᴇɴsɪs ᴘʜɪʟ. ᴇᴛ ᴘʜɪʟᴏʟ. ɢʀ. 219. l. 1 ὄμνυμι: ὑγίειαν. l. 2 θεούς τε. l. 5 δὲ: ἴσα γενήτησιν. l. 7 ποιεῖσθαι: εωυτέου. l. 8 τοῖς χρηίζουσι μανθάνειν. This is a unique variant. l. 9 ἀκρασιος, a reading which explains why the Latin translation of Nicolas of Regium (see p. 37) has *intemperantia*. l. 13 ἐπωφελείη. l. 14 ἐπιδηλήσει τε. l. 15 ποτε after οὐδενί. l. 16 ξυμβούλιον τοιόνδε. l. 17 τὸν ἐμὸν. l. 18 τὴν ἐμήν. l. 19 οὔτε for οὐδὲ: ληθιῶντας. l. 20 πράξιος. l. 21 εἰς: εἰσίω: εἰσελεύσομαι: ἐπωφελείη. l. 23 εὐανδρείων. l. 25 ἢ ἄνευ. l. 26 ἀνθρώπου: ἐκκαλέεσθαι. l. 30 εἰς: αἰεὶ. This manuscript differs from most *recentiores* in containing several variants that do not appear in M, V or R. They do not seem to be errors, and probably represent one of the many versions of *Oath* current in antiquity.

Hᴀᴜɴɪᴇɴsɪs ᴀɴᴛ. ꜰᴜɴᴅ. ʀᴇɢ. 224. l. 1 ὄμνυμι. l. 5 δὲ: ἴσα καὶ γενέτοισιν ἐμοῖσι. l. 7 ἑωυτέον: ἐπικρινέοιν: ἄρεσι. l. 14 ἐπιδηλήσει. l. 17 τὸν ἐμὸν. l. 18 τὴν ἐμὴν. l. 23 ἀνδρώων. In this manuscript *Oath* is followed by ἕτερος ὅρκος (αὐτὸν ἐν κ.τ.λ. See p. 57.)

Vᴏssɪᴀɴᴜs ꜰᴏʟ. 10. l. 1 ὄμνυμι. l. 5 ἡγήσασθαι μὲν: ἴσα γενέτοισιν ἐμοῖσιν. l. 6 μεταδίδωσιν. l. 7 ἑωυτέου: ἴσον. l. 14 ἐπιδηλήσει: εἴρξειν. l. 17 τὸν ἐμὸν. l. 18 τὴν ἐμήν. l. 22 φθορείης. l. 26 ἔξω. l. 30 εἰς: αἰεὶ.

I have made, or obtained, collations of nearly all the manuscripts not collated by Littré (and of two which he did collate), but I deeply regret that I have been unable to examine some two of them. They are late, but however late a manuscript may be, it is never safe to neglect it *unless we know that the scribe had access to no manuscript unknown to us.* Even Paris. 2146 and Holk. 282, which we know were copied from Vat. Gr. 276, are occasionally of use.

The early editors (e.g. Foes) sometimes quote from manuscripts now lost, but I have not noted any reading given by them which is not in at least one of our extant manuscripts.

A study of the later manuscripts impresses the reader with the completeness of the victory won by the M-V tradition. Nevertheless, besides the generally received text, we must consider:

(1) Vindobonensis philos. et philol. 219; (2) Scorialensis Σ II 5; (3) Ambrosianus B 113 sup. fol. 2; (4) the Christian oath.

The first has already been examined; it remains to discuss the other three.

THE OATH IN SCORIALENSIS Σ II 5

My colleague the Rev. H. J. Chaytor has visited the Escurial for me and collated Scorialensis Σ II 5 fol. 28ᵛ. In many respects it is the most interesting manuscript of *Oath*, because it combines, in an extraordinary manner, the pagan text with the Christian. Mr Chaytor's collation is as follows: l. 5 the first word is indecipherable, but looks like ὑτκσασθαι [ἡγήσασθαι?], followed by τὸν διδάξαντα. l. 7 τὸ ἐξ ἑωυτέου ἀδελφοῖσιν ἐμοῖσιν ἴσον. l. 10 μαθήσιος ἁπάσης. l. 11 διδάξαντος τὴν τέχνην ταύτην καὶ μαθηταῖσι. l. 13 χρῆσθαι (later hand χρήσομαι) πᾶσιν ἐπ'. l. 14 ἐπὶ κ.τ.λ. inserted by later hand. l. 16 γυναιξὶ. l. 19 ἀνδρ. ἐργ. πρή-ξεως. ll. 22–24 ἑκουσίης τε καὶ ἀκουσίης φθορίης τε καὶ τῆς ἄλλης λοιμώσεως ε (this letter in another hand)[1] ἀφρο-δισίων ἔργων ἐλευθέρων τε καὶ δούλων ἀπὸ ἀνδρ. τε καὶ γυν. σωμάτων. l. 29 ἐπαύρασθαί μοι γένοιτο καὶ βίου. l. 30 For παραβαίνοντι...τούτων, the MS reads εὐορκοῦντι μέν μοι εὖ ἐπιορκοῦντι δὲ τὰ ἐναντία τούτου.

This manuscript is quite unique. Besides the variants in ll. 7, 10, 11 and 19, which although unusual are slight, in several places the clauses follow closely the text of the Christian oath. As far as line 12 the readings are similar to those of the *textus receptus*, although ἐμοῖσιν ἴσον, μαθήσιος ἁπάσης and διδάξαντος τὴν τέχνην ταύτην are warnings that some other line of descent may have obtruded itself. At line 13 the suspicion becomes a certainty. There is πᾶσιν, as in Ambrosianus B 113 sup. and *omnibus* in the Latin version of Nicolas of Regium, while χρῆσθαι recalls the χρίσται of Bononiensis 3632 in the Christian oath. In l. 16 γυναιξὶ appears as in the Christian oath, while ll. 22–24 ἑκουσίης... σωμάτων are identical with the text of that form. In l. 29 ἐπαύρασθαί μοι γένοιτο καὶ βίου is a strange conflation of the pagan ἐπαύρασθαι καὶ βίου and the Christian βοηθός μοι γένοιτο ὁ θεὸς καὶ βίου. From this point onwards the text agrees with the Christian oath, except that the last word is τούτου, and not τουτέων.

[1] This ε must represent some contraction of καί.

The first part, then, follows the pagan oath, the latter the Christian. As it is the first part of the pagan oath which the Christian adapter omits, it is probable that Scorialensis Σ II 5 either:

(*a*) is a descendant of the form of the oath which the Christian adapter had in front of him;

or (*b*) represents an attempt by a later compiler to combine the two forms, the Christian and the pagan.

On the whole I should be inclined to give the preference to the view (*a*). There was probably in ancient times a form of *Oath* which gave us the Christian text by omissions, and Scorialensis Σ II 5 by additions such as the οὐ τεμέω clause.

In any case it is plain that in antiquity there were current many forms of the Hippocratic oath; that the *textus receptus*, or M-V tradition, has swamped the other forms seems to be a mere accident.

THE OATH IN AMBROS. B 113 SUP. (FOL. 2)

The Milan manuscript Ambrosianus B 113 sup. (fourteenth century) contains both pagan and Christian oath. The former is so different from the vulgate that I give here as accurate a transcription as I can make from the rotograph kindly sent to me by the Librarian of the Ambrosian Library. I was unable to see it until I had written my *Essay*, which I leave as I originally wrote it, in order that the reader may see how far my conclusions are confirmed by this strange manuscript. A few of its peculiarities are merely errors, but the majority show that our vulgate represents but one line of descent, and that probably not the best.

ΤΟΥ ΑΥΤΟΥ, Ο ΟΡΚΟΣ

ὄμνυμι ἀπόλλωνα ἰητρόν. καὶ ἀσκληπιόν. καὶ ⟨ὑγείαν.⟩[1] καὶ
πανάκειαν. καὶ θεοὺς ἅπαντάς τε καὶ πάσας, ἵστορας ποιεύμενος,
ἐπιτελέας ποιῆσαι κατὰ δύναμιν καὶ κρίσιν ἐμήν, ὅρκον τόνδε
καὶ ξυγγραφὴν τήνδε : ἡγήσασθαι πρῶτον τὸν διδάξαντά με
τέχνην τήνδε καὶ ξυγγραφὴν τήνδε, ἴσα γενέτῃσιν ἐμοῖσι. καὶ 5
βίου κοινώσασθαι, καὶ χρεῶν χρήζοντι, μελεδῶσι ποιήσασθαι·
καὶ γένους τοὺς ἐξ αὐτέου, ἀδελφοῖς ἴσον ἐπικρίνειν ἄρρεσιν· καὶ
διδάξω τὴν τέχνην ἣν χρήζωσι μανθάνειν, ἄνευ μισθοῦ καὶ ξυγ-
γραφῆς· παραγγελίης τὲ καὶ ἀκροήσιος καὶ τῆς λοιπῆς μαθήσιος,
πᾶσι μετάδοσιν ποιήσασθαι υἱοῖς τὲ ἐμοῖσι, καὶ τοῖσι τοῦ με 10
διδάξαντος· καὶ μαθητῇσι, ξυγγεγραμμένοισι νόμῳ ἰητρικῷ· ἄλλῳ
δὲ οὐδενί· διαιτήμασι πᾶσι κεχρῆσθαι κατὰ δύναμιν καὶ κρίσιν
ἐμήν, ἐπ᾽ ὠφελίῃ καμνόντων· ἐπὶ δόλοισι δὲ καὶ ἀδικίῃ, εἵρξειν
κατὰ γνώμην ἐμήν. οὐδὲν δὲ δώσω φάρμακον αἰτηθεὶς θανά-
σιμον· οὐδ᾽ ὑφηγήσομαι συμβουλίην τοιήνδε· οὐδὲ γυναικὶ φθόριον 15
παρέξω· ἁγνῶς δὲ καὶ ὁσίως διατηρήσω βίον ἐμὸν καὶ τέχνην
ἐμήν. οὔτ᾽ ἐμοῖσι δὲ οὔτ᾽ ἄλλοισιν ἐκχωρήσω ἀνδράσιν ἐργάτῃσιν

l. 3 Note the tense of ποιῆσαι. 4 Is πρῶτον a sign of deep-seated corruption?
5 Note τήνδε, not ταύτην. 5 καὶ ξυγγραφὴν τήνδε seems a mere repetition
of the same words above. 6 μελεδῶσι seems a mere mistake. 7 γένους
τοὺς seems a conflation of γένος τὸ and τοὺς. 8 τὴν τέχνην "the art," as often
in the Hippocratic writings for "medicine." 10 Note the addition of πᾶσι.
12 Note the reading κεχρῆσθαι. 13 ἐπὶ δόλοισι seems a very old variant for
ἐπὶ δηλήσει of the vulgate. 14 κατὰ γνώμην ἐμήν is not in the vulgate. 14 Note
the variant οὐδέν. 15, 16 γυναικὶ and παρέξω differ from the ordinary text.
17 οὔτ᾽ ἐμοῖσι κ.τ.λ. This is the most important variant. The writer evidently

[1] Omitted (I think through the photographer's error) in the rotograph.

πρήξιος τῆσδε. εἰς οἰκίην δὲ ἐὰν εἰσίω, ἐλεύσομαι ἐπ' ὠφελείῃ
καμνόντων. ἐκτὸς ἐὼν πάσης ἀδικίης καὶ φθορῆς τὲ τῆς ἄλλης·
καὶ ἀπὸ ἀφροδισίων ἔργων. καὶ ἐπὶ ἐλευθέρων καὶ δούλων καὶ ἐπὶ
ἀνδρώων καὶ γυναικείων σωμάτων. ὅσα δὲ ἐν θεραπείῃ ἢ ἴδω ἢ
5 ἀκούσω ἢ ἄνευ θεραπείης κατὰ βίον ἀνθρώπων, ἃ μὴ χρὴ ἔξω
λαλεύεσθαι, σιγήσομαι· ἄρρητα ἡγεύμενος εἶναι τὰ τοιαῦτα· ὅρκον
μὲν δὴ τόνδε ἐπιτελέα ποιέοντι καὶ μὴ ξυγχέοντι, εἴη ἐπεύρασθαι·
καὶ βίου καὶ τέχνης δοξαζομένῳ παρὰ πᾶσιν ἀνθρώποις εὖ τὸν
ἀεὶ χρόνον. ἐπιορκοῦντι δὲ καὶ παραβαίνοντι, τἀναντία τουτέων.

means, "I will not allow any subordinate, whether belonging to me or to others,
to perform this act" (i.e. abortion). πρήξιος τῆσδε is to be construed with
ἐκχωρήσω, and not with ἐργάτῃσιν. This reading clears away every difficulty
connected with this part of *Oath*. The operation-clause simply disappears,
and its place is taken by one meaning that all connivance at abortion is
forbidden. This is exactly the sense required by the context, and can hardly
fail to be the true reading, or a modification of it. It is still a puzzle how the
οὐ τεμέω clause arose, but it is at least remarkable that the new reading, like
the vulgate, begins with the letters οὐτεμ.   2 Note that the vulgate ἑκουσίης
is omitted.   8 The εὖ may be a mere mistake for εἰς. It may, however, be a
relic of the peculiar reading at this place in the Christian oath.

Finally I give the main conclusions which this remarkable
manuscript seems to indicate:

(1) The vulgate is not the only form of *Oath* current in
    ancient times.

(2) One form did not contain the operation-clause, but
    in its place one making more stringent the abortion-
    clause.

(3) The origin of the operation-clause is still obscure, but
    may be partly due to the first letters (οὐτεμ).

(4) Apart from the operation-clause, there are many peculiar readings, some of which (*e.g.* γυναιξὶ for γυναικὶ of the vulgate) suggest that this form of the text is connected with the Christian form. It is difficult, however, because of blunders, to decide whether this text is or is not generally superior to the M-V text.

CHRISTIAN OATH

TEXT

Ἐκ τοῦ κατὰ τὸν Ἱπποκράτεα ὅρκου καθ' ὅσον
οἷόν τε Χριστιανῷ ὀμόσαι.

The *titulus* appears in all three MSS. In Ambros. it is on the
preceding page. Ambros. has Ἱπποκράτην, and Bonon. κὰ θόσον
οἴονται Χριστιανῶν ὀμῶσαι.

Εὐλογητὸς ὁ θεὸς καὶ πατὴρ τοῦ κυρίου ἡμῶν Ἰησοῦ Χριστοῦ,
ὁ ὢν εὐλογητὸς εἰς τοὺς αἰῶνας, ὅτι οὐ ψεύδομαι. οὐ μολυνῶ
τὴν τῆς ἰατρικῆς τέχνης μάθησιν. οὐδὲ δώσω τινὶ αἰτηθεὶς φάρμακον θανάσιμον, οὐδὲ ὑφηγήσομαι ξυμβουλὴν τοιήνδε. ὁμοίως δὲ
5 οὐδὲ γυναικὶ δώσω φθόριον, ἄνωθέν τε ἢ κάτωθεν. ἀλλὰ διδάξω τὴν
τέχνην ταύτην, ἣν χρῇζωσιν μανθάνειν, ἄνευ φθόνου τε καὶ ξυγγραφῆς. καὶ διαιτήμασιν χρήσομαι ἐπ' ὠφελείης καμνόντων κατὰ
δύναμιν καὶ κρίσιν ἐμήν. καὶ ἁγνῶς καὶ ὁσίως διατηρήσω τέχνην
ἐμήν. ἐς οἰκίας ὁκόσας ἂν εἰσίω, εἰσελεύσομαι ἐπ' ὠφελείῃ καμνόντων,
10 ἐκτὸς ἐὼν πάσης ἀδικίης, ἑκουσίης τε καὶ ἀκουσίης, φθορίης τε

Urb. = Urbinas 64: Ambros. = Ambrosianus B 113 sup.: Bonon. = Bononiensis
3632. The last is not cruciform, and is difficult to read, containing many atrocious
misspellings. The parts peculiar to the Christian oath contain many non-ionic
forms, e.g. ὤν, ἰατρικῆς, λοιμώσεως, ἐνορκοῦντι. No attempt has been made to make
the spelling of the printed text consistent, as the compiler himself cannot have been so.

l. 2 μολύνω all MSS.   6 ἣν χρῆσιν χρήξουσιν μανθάνειν Urb.: ὡς ἔνι (query
ἔῃ or ἂν ᾖ) δέον καὶ χρῆζον καὶ ἁρμόζον Χριστιανοῖς μαθεῖν Ambros.: τῆς θέλοσιν
μάνθάνην Bonon.   7 Urb. and Ambros. omit χρήσομαι. Bonon. appears to have
χρίσται (χρῆσθαι?).   7 Perhaps ὠφελείῃ.   8 So Urb. and Bonon.: Ambros.
has κατὰ δύναμιν ἐμὴν καὶ κρίσιν ὀρθήν, κατὰ τὸ ἐγχωροῦν τῶ ἡμετέρω νῶ (gloss).
8 So Urb. and Ambros.: Bonon. has βίω τε καὶ τέχνην ἐμήν.   9 ὁκόσας Urb.
and Ambros.: ὁπόσας Bonon. After εἰσίω Urb. and Ambros. have ἢ, which may
have been written by a scribe who thought that εἰσελεύσομαι was an alternative
form for εἰσίω, or it possibly arose from the εἰ- following.   9 ὠφελεῖ Urb.:
ὠφελεία Ambros.: ὑφελίαν Bonon.   10 ἑκουσίοις Urb.

FROM THE OATH ACCORDING TO HIPPOCRATES
IN SO FAR AS A CHRISTIAN MAY SWEAR IT

Blessed be God the Father of our Lord Jesus Christ, who is blessed for ever and ever; I lie not.

I will bring no stain upon the learning of the medical art. Neither will I give poison to anybody though asked to do so, nor will I suggest such a plan. Similarly I will not give treatment[1] to women to cause abortion, treatment neither from above nor from below[2]. But I will teach this art, to those who require to learn it[3], without grudging and without an indenture. I will use treatment to help the sick according to my ability and judgment. And in purity and in holiness I will guard my art[4]. Into whatsoever houses I enter, I will do so to help the sick, keeping myself free from all wrongdoing, intentional or unintentional, tending to death or to

---

[1] φθόριον: sc. φάρμακον. The pagan oath has πεσσόν as the substantive.

[2] Not in pagan oath. The phrase was apparently added to meet the case of those who thought that they could obey the Hippocratic oath if they used other means than a pessary to produce abortion.

[3] The MSS vary here. I have translated Urb. 64, but Ambros. has "as is necessary, right and fitting for Christians to learn it," and Bonon. 3632 has "to those who wish to learn it."

[4] Bonon. 3632 has (as in pagan oath) "my life and my art." Note that in the next sentence even unintentional (ἀκουσίης) harm is forbidden. The doctor must not be criminally negligent. The word ἀκουσίης is not in the pagan oath, but occurs in the strange manuscript Scorialensis Σ II 5.

καὶ τῆς ἄλλης λοιμώσεως, καὶ ἀφροδισίων ἔργων, ἐλευθέρων τε καὶ
δούλων, ἀπὸ ἀνδρείων τε καὶ γυναικείων σωμάτων. ὅσα δ᾽ ἂν ἐν
θεραπείῃ ἢ ἴδω ἢ ἀκούσω, ἢ ἄνευ θεραπείης συγκαταβιῶν ἀνθρώποις, ἃ μὴ χρὴ ἔξω λαλῆσαι, σιγήσομαι, ἄρρητα ἡγεύμενος
5 εἶναι τὰ τοιαῦτα. ὅρκον μὲν οὖν μοι τόνδε ἐπιτελέα ποιέοντι καὶ
μὴ ξυγχέοντι, βοηθός μοι γένοιτο ὁ θεὸς καὶ βίου καὶ τέχνης,
δοξαζομένῳ παρὰ πᾶσιν ἀνθρώποισιν ἐς τὸν ἀεὶ χρόνον. εὐορκοῦντι μέν μοι εὖ· ἐπιορκοῦντι δὲ τὰ ἐναντία τουτέων.

l. 2 ἀνδρίων Urb.: ἀνδρώων Ambros.: ἀνδρὶον Bonon.   3 συγκαταβίων
ἀνῶν Urb.: συγκατα ἀνῶν Ambros.: κατὰ βίο ἀνῶν Bonon. (as in pagan oath).
4 λαλεῖσαι Urb.: λαλῆσαι Ambros.: λαλῆσται (?) Bonon. Perhaps λαλεῖσθαι.
6 Urb. seems to read ξυχέοντι, Bonon. σιχέοντι. τέχνης: So Urb. and Ambros.:
Bonon. adds ὁδιγός (i.e. ὁδηγός).   8 Instead of εὐορκοῦντι...δὲ Bonon. has
παραβένοντι δὲ καὶ ἐπιορκοῦντι. Urb. seems to punctuate before εὖ.   8 τοῦ
τέλος (or τέλους) Urb.: τοῦ τέλους Ambros.: τοῦ τέων Bonon. Apparently a
"portmanteau" of τουτέων and τὸ τέλος.

injury, and from fornication with bond or free, man or woman. Whatsoever in the course of practice I see or hear (or outside my practice in social intercourse) that ought not to be published abroad, I will not divulge, but consider such things to be holy secrets. Now if I keep this oath and break it not, may God be my helper in my life and art[1], and may I be honoured among all men for all time. If I keep faith, well[2]; but if I forswear myself may the opposite befall me[3].

---

[1] Bonon. 3632 has "may God be my helper and guide in my life and art."

[2] This sentence is not in Bonon. 3632, which has, however (as in the pagan oath), "but if I transgress and forswear myself."

[3] I think the τέλους (or τέλος) of Urb. and Ambros. to be a mere blunder.

CHRISTIAN OATH IN AMBROSIANUS B 113 SUP.

Εὐλογητὸς ὁ θς καὶ πηρ τοῦ κυ
ἡμῶν ιυ χυ· ὁ ὢν εὐλογητὸς
εἰς τοὺς αἰῶνας, ὅτι οὐ τεθειδῆ.
ὁμολογῶ τὴν τῆς ἰατρικῆς
τέχνης μάθησιν. οὐδὲ δώσω
τινὰ τῆς ἧς. φάρμακον θανάσιμον. οὐδὲ ὑφηγήσομαι ξυμ-
βουλην τοίην δέ· ὁμοίως δὲ, οὐδὲ
γυναικὶ δώσω φθόριον. ἁγνῶς δὲ
τηρήσω κατὰ τῶν. ἀλλὰ δὴ δείξω
τὴν τέχνην ταύτην, ὡς ἐπὶ δίον καὶ χρήσιμον καὶ ἀρμόδιον χρησθαι
μαθεῖν, ἀνὰ φθόνου τε καὶ ξυγγραφῆς καὶ διδασκαλίης, ἐπὶ
ὠφελείης καμνόντων. κατὰ δύναμιν ἐμὴν καὶ κρίσιν ὀρθήν,
κατὰ τὸ ὀχυρὸν τῶν ἑτέρων· καὶ ἁγνῶς καὶ ὁσίως διατηρήσω τέχνην ἐμήν· ἐς οἰκίας ὁκόσας ἂν εἰσίω ἢ εἰσελεύσομαι,
ἐπὶ ὠφελείᾳ καμνόντων. ἐκτὸς
ἐὼν, πάσης ἀδικίης, ἑκουσίης
καὶ ἀκουσίης. φθορίης τε, καὶ
ἀμπελοργίης καὶ ἀφροδισί-
ων ἔργων. ἐλευθέρων τε καὶ δούλων,
ἀπὸ ἀνδρῶν τε καὶ γυναικείων
σωμάτων. ὅσα ἂν ἐν θεραπείᾳ
ἢ ἴδω ἢ ἀκούσω ἢ ἄνευ θεραπείης
σιγήσομαι ἄξων, ἀλλ' εἴ χρη
ἐξολαλήσαι, σιγήσομαι ἄρρητα
ἡγούμενος εἶναι τὰ τοιαῦτα. ὅρκον μὲν οὖν μοι τόνδε ἐπιτελέα ποιέοντι καὶ μὴ ξυγχέοντι, βοηθός μοι γένοιτο ὁ θς. καὶ βίου
καὶ τέχνης. δοξαζομένω παρὰ πᾶσιν ἀνθρώποισιν, εἰς τὸν ἀεὶ
χρόνον. δ' ὅρκω ἡμέν μοι, δ' ἐπιορκοῦντι δὲ, τὰ
ἐναντία τούτέοι.

To the facsimiles of Urbinas 64 and Ambrosianus B 113 sup. I append a transcription of Bononiensis 3632. It is very badly written and spelt, and in places I am in doubt as to the exact spelling.

ἐκ τοῦ κατὰ τὸν Ἱπποκράτην(?) ὅρκου κὰ θόσον οἴονται Χριστιανῶν ὀμῶσαι:—

Εὐλογητὸς ὁ θεὸς καὶ πατήρ του κυρίου ἡμῶν γισου[1] Χριστού ὁ ὢν εὐλογητος ἧς τοὺς αιῶνας ὃ τι ου ψεύδομαι. οὐ μολύνω τὴν τῆς ἰατρικῆς τέχνην μάθισην· οὐδὲ δόσω τηνῆς᾿ αἰτιθείς φάρμακον θανάσιμον· οὔτε οὐφυγήσωμαι συμβουλὴν τιάνδε· ὁμίος δὲ οὐδὲ γυνεξὴ δόσω φθόρειον· ἀνοθέν ται ἢ κάτοθεν· ἀλα διδάξο τὴν τέχνην ταύτην, τῆς θέλοσιν μὰνθάνην· ἄνευ θόνου τε ἢ σηγραφῆς. καὶ διέτημασι χρίσται πάσην ἐπόφελιαν καμνόντων· κατὰ δύναμιν καὶ κρίσιν ἐμὴν· καὶ ἀγνὸς καὶ ὅσιος διατυρίσω βίω τε καὶ τέχνην ἐμὴν. ἧς ἰκίας δὲ ὁπόσας ἂν ἠσίω· εἰσελεύσομαι ἐπόφελιαν κὰμνόντων· ἐκτὸς ἐῶ πάσης ἀδικίας ἑκουσίας τε καὶ ἀκουσίας· φθόριας ται. καὶ τῆς ἄλοις λυμώσαιος· καὶ ἀφρόδισιον ἔργον· ἐλεύθερόν τε καὶ δούλων. ἀπὸ ἀνδρίον ται καὶ δούλον· καὶ γυναικίον σομάτων. ὀκόσα δὲ ἐν θέραπια εἰ ἤδω· εἰ ἀκούσω· ἢ ἄνευ θεραπίας κατὰ βίο ἀνθρώπον, ἃ μὴ χρεὶ ἐξω λαλήσται συγήσωμαι· ἄρρητα υγεύμενος ἦναι τα τιαύτα· ὅρκον δέ μι τόνδε ἐπιτελή πιοῦντι, καὶ μυ συγχέοντι[2]· βοηθὸς μι γένητο ὁ θεὸς καὶ βίου καὶ τέχνης ὀδιγός. δοξαζομένω παρα πάσιν ἀνθρώποις· ἧς τὸν ἀεὶ χρῶνον. παραβένοντι δὲ καὶ ἐπιορκοῦντι, τἀνἀντια τοῦ τέων.

---

[1] I cannot decipher the first letter; it has the appearance of the English y.
[2] Perhaps σιχέοντι.

TRANSLATIONS

ARABIC

Oath passed through Syriac into Arabic, and a version is found in the *Lives of Physicians* written by Ibn abi Usaybia, who died in 1269. His Arabic translation, therefore, probably represents a Greek text some centuries earlier than this date. Through the kindness of Professor E. G. Browne and of Mr M. Z. Siddiqui I am able to give both a text and a translation of the Arabic.

The writer prefixes to his version a very reasonable account of the origin of *Oath*. He says that when it was found necessary to admit outsiders into the hereditary schools of Greek medicine, Hippocrates administered an oath, in order to secure candidates of a suitable character.

هذه نسخة العهد الذي وضَعه ابقراط

قال ابقراط اتّي أُقسِمُ بالله ربّ الحياة و الموت و واهب الصَحّة
و خالق الشّفاء و كلّ علاجٍ، و أُقسِمُ بـاسقلييـيوس، و أُقسِمُ بـاولياء
الله مِنَ الرجال و النساء جميعاً، و أُشهِدُهم جميعاً، على أتّي أفي
بهذه اليمين و هذا الشرط،

و أرىٰ أنّ المعلّمَ لي هذه الصناعة بمنزلة آبائي، و أُواسيه في معاشي،
و اذا احتاجَ الى مالٍ واسيتُه و واصلتُه من مالي، و أمّا الجنسُ المتناسلُ منه
فأرىٰ أنّه مساوٍ لاخُوتي، و أُعلّمُهم هذه الصناعة انِ احتاجوا الى
تعلّمِها بغير أجرةٍ و لا شرطٍ، و أشركُ اولادي و اولادَ المعلّمِ لي و
التلاميذَ الّذين كُتبّ عليهِم الشرطُ و أُحلفوا بالناموس الطبّي في
الوصايا و العلومِ و سائرِ ما في الصناعة، و أمّا غيرُ هؤلا فلا افعل
به ذلك،

و اقصد في جميع التدبير بقدر طاقتي منفعةَ المرضىٰ، و أمّا الاشياء
الّتي تَضُرُّ بهم و تدني منهم بالجور عليهِم فامنعُ منها بحسب رائي، و
لا أُعطي اذا طلب مني دواءً قتّالاً، و لا أُشيرُ ايضاً بمثل هذه المشورة،
و كذلك ايضاً لا أرىٰ أن ادنى من النسوة فرزجةً تسقط الجنين،
و أَحفظُ نفسي في تدبيري و صنا عتي على الزكاء و الطهارة، و لا
أَشقّ ايضاً عمّن في مثانته حجارةٌ، لكن أَترك ذلك الى مَن كانت

THE TEXT OF THE COVENANT LAID DOWN
BY HIPPOCRATES

Hippocrates said: I swear in the name of God, the Master of life and death, the Giver of health and Creator of healing and of every treatment, and I swear in the name of Aesculapius, and of all the holy ones of God, male and female, and I call them to witness, that I will fulfil this oath and these conditions. I will regard my teacher in this art as my father, I will share with him my means of livelihood, and I will make him my partner in my wealth, and I will give him my wealth whenever he may be in need of it.

As for his descendants, I regard them as my brothers, and I will teach them this art without any remuneration or condition, should they desire to learn it. And I associate together (*i.e.* regard as equal), in the injunctions and in the sciences and in all else contained in the art, my own children, the children of my teacher, and the disciples on whom the oath (or covenant) has been imposed, and who have sworn to observe the medical code of honour. And I will not do so for any other than these.

In all my treatment I will strive so far as lies in my power for the benefit of the patients. And I will restrain myself from things which are injurious to them, or are likely in my opinion to do them harm. And I will not give them any poisonous drug if they ask for it, nor will I advise them thus. Nor will I contemplate administering any pessary which may cause abortion. And in my treatment and in the

حرفته هذا العملُ، و كلُّ المنازل الّتي ادخلُها انّما ادخل اليها
لمنفعةِ المرضىٰ و انا بحالٍ خارجةٍ عن كلّ جورٍ و ظلمٍ و فسادٍ
اراديٍّ مقصودٍ اليه في سائرِ الاشياء و في الجماع للنساء و الرجالِ
الاحرارِ منهم و العبيد،

و امّا الاشياءُ الّتي اُعاينُها في اوقاتِ علاجِ المرض، او اسمعها، او
في غير اوقاتِ علاجهم في تصرّفِ النّاس من الاشياء الّتي لا ينطق
بها خارجاً فامسك عنها و ارىٰ انّ مثالها لا ينطق به،

فَمَنْ اكملَ هذه اليمينَ و لم يفسد منها شيئاً كانَ له اَن يكملَ
تدبيره و صناعته على افضلِ الاحوال و اجلها و اَنْ يحمده جميعُ
الناس فيما ياتي من الزّمانِ دائماً و مَنْ تجاوَز ذلكَ كانَ بضدّه،

Vol. I, p. 25. Cairo, 1882.

practice of my art I will keep myself pure and holy. And I will not operate on those who have stone in the bladder; rather I will leave it for those whose profession it is. And I will enter every abode into which I may go only for the benefit of the sick, being in a state devoid of (all deliberate intention of) wrong-doing, injustice, mischief-making, such as might be intended in other transactions, or in respect of sexual relations with woman or man, whether free or slaves.

And as for the things which I may see or hear during the time of treating the sick, or at times other than those in which I am so engaged, about such behaviour of men as should not be talked of outside, I will keep silence, considering that such things should not be discussed.

He who fulfils this oath and does not violate any part of it, to him will it be granted to carry out his treatment and his art under the most excellent and favourable conditions, and to be praised by all men in future for ever; while the contrary will be the portion of him who transgresses it.

LATIN

Two Latin translations of *Oath* are to be found in extant manuscripts[1], but they are rather disappointing. Professor Rostagno has sent me a transcription of Laurentianus 73, 40, fol. 108[2] (said by Diels to be a manuscript of the thirteenth century[3]), the *titulus* of which is "Hipocratis ius iurandum incipit feliciter per N. Perotum ex greco traductum." The text is the same as that found in the Leyden manuscript, B. P. L 156, Bernensis 531 fol. 111ᵛ, Vindobonensis 4772 fol. 62ᵛ and 63ʳ, and Basileensis E III 15 fol. 258[4].

This version is ascribed to N. Perotti in the little book, printed at Basle in 1538, entitled Γαλήνου περὶ κράσεων βιβλία τρία κ.τ.λ. pp. 138, 139.

> Leyden B. P. L 156 = L.
> Laurentianus 73, 40 = F.
> Bernensis 531 = B.
> Vindobonensis 4772 = V.
> Basileensis E III 15 = Ba.

---

[1] See H. Diels, *Die Handschriften der antiken Ärzte*, 1 Teil, p. 18, where detailed references to eight Latin manuscripts are given.

[2] The other manuscripts I have collated from rotographs, except V, a transcription of which has been sent to me by Dr Karl Mras, of Vienna.

[3] The part containing *Oath* is, so Professor Rostagno tells me, some two hundred years later than the rest of the manuscript.

[4] The version is ascribed in Vindobonensis 4772 to Petrus Paulus Vergerius (1349—1428), while Perotti lived from 1430 to 1480. The authorship is therefore uncertain, but the Latin appears mediaeval.

Testor Apollinem medicum et Aesculapium, Hygiamque
et Panaceam, Aesculapii filias, et deos ac deas omnes, me,
quantum in me erit et quantum ingenium meum valebit,
haec omnia observaturum quae hoc iureiurando atque his
tabellis continentur. tributurum me praeceptori meo a quo 5
hanc artem edoctus sum non minus quam parenti a quo
sum genitus; vitam cum eo communicaturum; res omnes
quas illi necessarias esse intellegam pro viribus meis sub-
ministraturum; progeniem eius fratrum loco habiturum;
hanc artem sine mercede et sine pactionibus edocturum. 10
praecepta omnia libere et fideliter traditurum meis et prae-
ceptoris mei liberis, ceterisque discipulis qui se legibus
medicinae astrinxerint atque iurati fuerint, alii praeterea
nemini. in curandis aegrotis pro viribus et pro ingenio meo
rebus necessariis usurum, nemini aegritudinem dilaturum, 15
nihil per iniuriam facturum. rogatum mortale venenum
nemini daturum, neque id cuiquam consulturum. neque
praegnanti mulieri ad interficiendum conceptum fetum
potionem porrecturum. vitam meam atque artem meam
puram atque integram servaturum. laborantis lapillo haud- 20
quaquam excisurum, sed expertis eius artis hoc negotium
permissurum. quamcumque domum ingressus fuero, dum-
taxat liberandis aegrotis operam daturum; omnem iniuriam,
omnem corruptelam, omne genus turpitudinis, res etiam

venereas sponte mea evitaturum, sive muliebria corpora
curavero sive virilia, sive hominis liberi, sive servi. quae
inter curandum vel videro vel audivero, vel etiam extra
curam in vita hominum cognovero, quae reticenda esse
5 intellegam, nemini aperturum, sed intemeratam taciturni-
tatem servaturum. praesens igitur iusiurandum integre atque
incorrupte servanti mihi omnia tam in vita quam in arte
mea prospera feliciaque succedant, et gloria in aeternum
parata sit; transgredienti vero atque periuro contraria omnia
10 eveniant.

1. 1 *curaturum* F. 2 *sive* before *hominis* omitted by B, Ba. *et* for *quae* F.
4 *cognovero* omitted by Ba: *curavero* B. *recitanda* F. 5 *intemeritatem*
taciturnitatemque B, Ba. 7 *morte* L, B, Ba. 9 *parta* F, B, Ba. 10 L. adds
τέλως (*sic*).

A more literal and, apparently, an earlier version is found
in Neapolitanus VIII D 25 fol. 84, the date of which is
1380 A.D., and in Matritensis 1978 (once L 60) fol. 96, a
manuscript of roughly the same age.

The version is attributed in the Naples manuscript to
Nicolas of Regium. I have done my best to reconstruct the
original, giving variants wherever there is any reasonable
doubt about the true reading.

Neapolitanus VIII D 25 = N.
Matritensis 1978 = M.

Iuro per Apollinem medicum et Sanitiam et Remediatiam
et deos universos et universas, scitores faciens, perficiam
secundum possibilitatem et actionem et iudicium meum
iuramentum hoc et conscriptionem istam. eum qui docuit
me artem hanc introducere inter meos, et communicare in 5
vita, et in quo indiget dationem facere, et genus quod ab ipso
fratribus aequale iudicare † eligam.† et docebo artem hanc
eos qui indigent discere absque pretio et conscriptione, et
† delusione et intemperantia † et de reliqua universa dis-
ciplina traditionem facere filiis meis et eius qui me docuit 10
et edoctis † et temperatis † et iuratis legi medicinali, alii
autem nulli. dietationibusque utar omnibus iuvamento
laborantium secundum possibilitatem et iudicium meum,
et de † incusatione † et iniustitia prohibebor. neque dabo
ulli farmacum rogatus mortale, neque narrabo consilium 15
tale. similiter autem neque mulieri pessarium corruptivum
dabo. pure vero et sancte servabo vitam meam et artem
meam. non incidam autem neque lapiditatem patientes, sed
dimittam hoc opus hominibus huius operationis. ad domos

1. 1 *sanativam* M. 2 *sicores* M. 3 The Greek text has nothing to corre-
spond to *actionem*. 4 Before *eum* M has *prosequi*. 7 *indicare* N. 7 Possibly the
translator read αἱρήσω for our ἄρρεσι. 9 Apparently *de lusione*. Perhaps παραγγελίης τε καὶ ἀκροήσιος was misread παιγνίης τε καὶ ἀκρασίης. See p. 14 and p. 15.
11 M appears to read *temperantius*. *Edoctis* may well represent μαθηρῆσι, but συγγεγραμμένοις should have been translated *conscriptis*, as συγγραφή is rendered by *con-
scriptio*. 11 N has *legis*. 12 M has *in iuramento*. 14 M has *demensatione* for *de
incusatione*. The Greek is ἐπὶ δηλήσει. Perhaps *de destructione*. The translator, however, may have written *incuratione*, as he did not hesitate to coin words (*scitores*). 18 M
has *inlapidenitatem*, N *neque lapideitatem*. A translator's coinage in any case.
19 M has *operis* for *operationis*.

autem ad quotcumque ivero, ibo ad utilitatem eorum qui
laborant, absque omni iniustitia spontanea et corruptiva
alia, et venereorum operum in † mulieribus corporibus †,
liberorum et servorum. ea vero quae in cura videro aut
5 audivero, vel etiam absque cura de vitis hominum, quae non
sit conveniens loqui extra, tacebo, ceu neque videre ea
putans. iuramentum itaque meum et conscriptionem hanc
qui perfectum facit et non confringit erit diligibilis ut
augeatur et in vita et arte honorandus ab omnibus hominibus
10 in sempiterno tempore, transgredienti autem et † deieranti †
contraria horum.

l. 3 N has *mulioribus*. Something appears to have been left out, as there is nothing
to represent ἀνδρείων. 4 M omits *vero*. 7 M has *eciam* for *itaque*. 8 Note that
the Latin here changes to the third person. No Greek manuscript shows this
peculiarity, but it appears in the Arabic. 10 M has *degeranti*. The right reading
would be *peieranti*.

ESSAY

The document called "the Hippocratic oath" presents many problems the answers to which seem to be lost for ever. At the same time it sends out tiny rays of light which illumine for a moment some of the dark places of history, showing us how great our ignorance is by the very scantiness of the information it affords. Nevertheless it will always interest the historian of ethics as well as the professional physician. Here we have an early record of those noble rules of conduct, loyal obedience to which has raised the art of medicine to the high position it now holds. Puzzling doubts and tantalising uncertainties cannot obliterate this precious truth. The rules contained in *Oath*, however, do not necessarily apply to everybody, but only to medical men. Abortion, for example, though doctors are forbidden to cause it, was possibly not condemned in all cases.

The first certain reference to *Oath* is in the preface of Scribonius Largus[1], a medical writer living in the reign of Claudius. He says that Hippocrates, "the founder of our profession," began his instruction with an oath, in which the practice of abortion was forbidden. Erotian[2], a lexicographer of the time of Nero, mentions an oath among the genuine

---

[1] Helmreich, p. 2: Hippocrates, conditor nostrae professionis, initia disciplinae ab iureiurando tradidit, in quo sanctum est, ne praegnati quidem medicamentum, quo conceptum excutitur, aut detur aut demonstretur a quoquam medico, longe praeformans animos discentium ad humanitatem.

[2] Nachmanson, p. 9.

works of Hippocrates, and there are later references in Jerome[1], Gregory Nazianzen[2] and Suidas[3].

It is likely, however, that there is a much earlier allusion to *Oath* in the *Thesmophoriazusae* of Aristophanes. In that comedy Euripides is asked by his kinsman Mnesilochus to swear to help him, and the following dialogue takes place[4]:

> EUR. I swear then by aether, abode of Zeus.
> MNE. Why, rather than by the community of Hippocrates?
> EUR. I swear then by all the gods wholesale.

The scholiast thinks that the reference is to an Athenian Hippocrates notorious for the silliness of his family, but this explanation certainly appears forced and unnatural[5], and Aristophanes probably had in mind the opening words of *Oath*, with their comprehensive συνοικία of divinities. So an Hippocratic oath may have been known as early as 400 B.C.

It is indeed hard to believe that the nucleus, at least, of

---

[1] *Epist.* 52: Migne, *Patr. Lat.* 22, col. 539. This passage will be discussed later.

[2] Migne, *Patr. Gr.* 35, col. 767.

[3] *S.v.* Hippocrates.

[4] Ll. 272–274:

> ΕΥ. ὄμνυμι τοίνυν αἰθέρ' οἴκησιν Διός.
> ΜΝ. τί μᾶλλον ἢ τὴν Ἱπποκράτους ξυνοικίαν;
> ΕΥ. ὄμνυμι τοίνυν πάντας ἄρδην τοὺς θεούς.

[5] So Pétrequin, p. 172, note 1, who adopts the view advanced by D. Triller in the eighteenth century. Littré does not see an allusion to the Hippocratic oath. There is a reference to the Athenian Hippocrates and his sons in *Clouds* 1001. This evidence can be used either way. It may be said that the two references are probably to the same person; or, again, that the scholiast has wrongly identified the Hippocrates of the *Clouds* with the Hippocrates of the *Thesmophoriazusae*. But between the plays was an interval of eleven years (422–411 B.C.). Surely a topical allusion cannot enjoy such a long life.

Oath does not go back to the "great" Hippocrates himself. Nobody else is more likely to have framed such a fine guide to medical morality.

The two versions of *Oath*, pagan and Christian, and the peculiar variants they present, particularly the variants of the Christian oath, suggest that the document had a wide circulation, and that the text was far from being stereotyped. There are, for instance, serious difficulties connected with the operation-clause, which can be explained only by regarding it as an interpolation due to special circumstances of place or of time. The pagan text, the usual form of which goes back no further than the common ancestor of M and V, may have admitted, and probably did admit, before the time of this common ancestor, variations which are now lost[1]. This opinion is perhaps corroborated by the reference to *Oath* in Jerome. He says that Hippocrates forced his pupils, by an oath, to adopt certain rules of conduct with regard to "silence, speech, gait, manner and character"[2]. There is a clause in *Oath* dealing with silence, but there is nothing in the extan forms which touches on either *incessus* or *habitus*. We are forced to the conclusion that either Jerome has inadvertently included under the term *sacramentum* rules of conduct which appear, not in *Oath*, but in *Precepts* or in *Decorum*, the two

---

[1] See the text of Ambrosianus B 113 sup. on p. 19, which I saw after writing the above, and the collation of Scorialensis Σ II 5 given on p. 17.

[2] *Ep.* 52: Migne, *Patr. Lat.* 22, col. 539: Hippocrates adiurat discipulos suos, antequam doceat, et in verba sua iurare compellit, extorquet sacramento silentium, sermonem, incessum, habitum, moresque praescribit.

works of the Hippocratic Collection which, after *Oath*, give us most information about ancient medical etiquette, or else that in early Christian times there were forms of *Oath* which included references to *incessus* and *habitus*. Of the two suppositions the second is perhaps the more likely. It is therefore probable, if not certain, that the two surviving forms are but the remains of what was once a far more numerous and far more varied series of documents. It is unfortunate that none of our first-class manuscripts contains *Oath*. Had it appeared in A or in θ we should probably have known much more about its history and meaning.

Even though we admit the antiquity of *Oath*, we are still confronted with the difficult problem of its nature. What was its sanction? Did any penalties follow the breaking of it? Did all medical students swear it, or only those belonging to a community or guild? Was it ever actually administered, or was it a mere counsel of perfection held up to the respectful admiration of practitioners?

It is fairly certain that a doctor who did not follow this oath was not punished unless he sinned against the laws of the State. The writer of the quaint little piece called *Law*[1], one of the most interesting tractates in the Hippocratic Collection, complains that the only penalty to which the erring doctor was subject was dishonour, and this, he adds, was no punishment to those who were "compacted of it"[2].

---

[1] Ch. I: πρόστιμον γὰρ ἰητρικῆς μούνης ἐν τῇσι πόλεσιν οὐδὲν ὥρισται, πλὴν ἀδοξίης. αὕτη δὲ οὐ τιτρώσκει τοὺς ἐξ αὐτῆς συγκειμένους.

[2] The writer of *Nature of the Child* (Littré VII 490) narrates unblushingly how

This slackness of the discipline exercised by the State accounts for the stringency and solemnity of *Oath*. In days when there was no General Medical Council it was necessary to make every possible appeal to religious scruples and to the moral sense.

One clause in *Oath* expressly states that a person subscribing to it must give special favours to his teacher and his family, and communicate the secrets of the medical craft only to his sons, to the sons of his teacher, and to adopted outsiders who have sworn allegiance to "the physicians' Law"[1]. We have here some of the essential elements of a guild or trade union.

he attempted to produce an abortion in a singularly disgusting manner. Such violations of the spirit of *Oath* while the letter was kept possibly induced the writer of the Christian oath to be more explicit. See p. 52.

[1] This passage contains many linguistic peculiarities. In the first place ἴστωρ in the sense of "witness" (*cf.* ἴστω Ζεύς) is poetic. Then the aorists ἡγήσασθαι etc. are strange, not in themselves, but because of their combination with ἐπικρινεῖν and διδάξειν. The manuscript authority in favour of the aorists is overwhelming; and for this reason, and also because they may represent a conflation of two readings, one with futures and one with aorists, I have left them in the text. Again γενέτῃσι ("parents" or "ancestors") is a poetic word which aroused the curiosity of the scholiast (Littré IV p. 628). Some manuscripts read ἴσα καὶ γενέτῃσιν ἐμοῖσιν, an hexameter ending which suggests that this part of *Oath* may originally have been written in verse. Compare the metrical oath quoted on p. 57. Then again the reflexive form ἑωυτέου, given by many of the manuscripts I have examined, and the poetic forms ἴσα, ἴσον given by several, are very strange. Why should the epithet ἄρρεσι be attached to ἀδελφοῖς? It seems quite otiose. Finally I feel sure that all scholars will consider the division of instruction into παραγγελίη, ἀκρόησις and ἡ λοιπὴ μάθησις, curious and unusual. Is it a coincidence that these peculiarities occur at the beginning of *Oath*, where the apprentice binds himself to support a sort of guild? Is not the language "liturgical'?

Now Galen knew nothing about *Oath*; at any rate he never alludes to it. Nevertheless it is most interesting that he tells us[1] how ancient physicians comprised a "clan of the Asclepiadae" (γένος Ἀσκληπιαδῶν) who taught their sons practical anatomy, and how they in their turn transmitted it verbally in great perfection. After a time the Asclepiadae began to take adult pupils from outside; but these transmitted the art much less perfectly.

It is well known that at least from the time of Theognis[2] a medical man was often called an "Asclepiad," just as nowadays any qualified practitioner is by courtesy styled a "doctor." Nevertheless, we cannot doubt the assertion that there was an exclusive family of physicians, who called themselves Asclepiads and laid claim to superior knowledge and skill. Probably the family had ceased to exist before the time of Galen.

The question naturally arises whether *Oath* was the test required before an outsider became a member by adoption of this γένος Ἀσκληπιαδῶν. Many modern scholars, including Littré, Jowett and Gomperz, assume that it was, and this view is at least not inconsistent with the account of the Asclepiadae given by Galen. To say more than this is perhaps illegitimate.

It should be noticed that all the linguistic peculiarities[3]

---

[1] Kühn II 281. Compare Plato *Laws* IV 720 B: τούς τε αὐτῶν διδάσκουσι παῖδας.

[2] Ll. 432–434. Other references are Galen (Kühn) X 4; XIII 273; XIV 676; Plato *Republic* 405, 406; *Protagoras* 311 B; Lucian *Lexiphanes* 4.

[3] γενέτῃσιν, ἀδελφοῖς ἄρρεσι etc. See p. 43.

of *Oath* occur in the passage that binds the apprentice to his guild. The reader is asked to bear this in mind when reading the paragraphs that follow.

It is clear that *Oath* binds the apprentice to a society approximating to a guild or trade union; can we go further, and say that this society was a secret one? *Oath* itself affords us no evidence beyond the first few clauses, but other Hippocratic works lend some plausibility to this view.

All the θίασοι of which we know were associated with the cult of some deity or deities, and there is no trace of such a cult in the Hippocratic writings. Moreover, a cult of Asclepius would give us as the name of its members Ἀσκλη-πιασταί, not Ἀσκληπιάδαι. But there is reason to suppose that certain societies, not θίασοι, held meetings, with addresses or lectures, from which outsiders were excluded. The Pythagoreans perhaps held such meetings.

Two treatises in the Hippocratic Collection, *Precepts* and *Decorum*, are very like addresses to secret societies. They seem strangely familiar to Masons of high degree. The language is extremely quaint, and in many parts very obscure, as though the writer did not wish to be understood[1] by outsiders unfamiliar with the liturgy and ritual of the society. Sometimes the meaning quite escapes us, and we are led to suppose that the lecturer jotted down notes which he expounded to his audience orally. *Decorum* closes with an

---

[1] Of course the obscurity may be due to the perverted taste which is at its worst in Lycophron. Both *Precepts* and *Decorum* are late.

appeal to acquire certain knowledge, "to keep it safe and to pass it on."

Law is an address to young students delivered at the commencement of their medical course. It ends thus:

"But holy things are shown to holy men. The profane may not be shown them until they have been initiated into the rites of science"[1].

In *Precepts*[2] a genuine physician of sound principles is styled ἠδελφισμένος, which can only mean "one who has been made a brother"—surely a brother of a fraternity or guild.

Such in brief is the evidence. It would be overwhelming to anyone acquainted with secret societies, were it not for the objection that θίασοι were always connected with religious cults[3].

Custom and convenience, to say nothing of the human conscience, would sooner or later lay down most of the rules of conduct comprised in *Oath*, but there is one sentence which appears strange, and no solution of the problem hitherto offered seems entirely adequate. I refer to the words οὐ τεμέω δὲ οὐδὲ μὴν λιθιῶντας, ἐκχωρήσω δὲ ἐργάτῃσιν ἀνδράσι πρήξιος τῆσδε. Grammatically, the first clause of this sentence may mean:

---

[1] τὰ δὲ ἱερὰ ἐόντα πρήγματα ἱεροῖσιν ἀνθρώποισι δείκνυται· βεβήλοισι δὲ οὐ θέμις, πρὶν ἢ τελεσθῶσιν ὀργίοισιν ἐπιστήμης. The sentence is full of the language of secret societies (ἱερά, δείκνυται, βεβήλοισι, τελεσθῶσιν, ὀργίοισιν), and unless it is entirely metaphorical can imply only that the applicants must be initiated before they can be "shown" any more. Note also that in *Oath* reference is made to esoteric teaching (ἀκρόησιος).

[2] Chap. v.   [3] See my *Hippocrates* vol. II pp. 272–276 and 333–336.

(1) "As to operating, I, furthermore, will not operate for stone."

(2) "Moreover, I will not operate, not even for stone."

Between the two interpretations, linguistically, there is but little to choose, except that, if (2) be correct, it would be usual for μὴν to occur a little earlier.

As to the sense, however, there is a great difference between (1) "I will not operate," and (2) "I will not operate for stone." The commentators[1] adopt the second of these two interpretations. The question at once arises whether the operation for stone was ever forbidden by custom or etiquette, and on this point antiquity is perplexingly silent. The operation is often described, for example by Celsus, but no writer positively states that he has performed it himself. As to operations generally, the Hippocratic writers performed them without fear or scruple. The only light thrown on this dark problem is the statement of Galen[2] that when he came to Rome operations were performed by a special class whom he calls "surgeons" (χειρουργοί).

Moreover, whether the clause refers to operations in general or to cutting for stone in particular, it is strangely out of place in its context. Before it and after it are clauses dealing with moral offences; among these occurs this sentence relating to a delicate point of medical etiquette. Accordingly many scholars, Gomperz and Reinhold among them, have

---

[1] The editors in *Kleine Texte* postulate a lacuna between δὲ and οὐδὲ.

[2] Kühn I 454, 455: διατρίψας δ' ἐν Ῥώμῃ τὰ πλεῖστα τῷ τῆς πόλεως ἔθει συνηκολούθησα, παραχωρήσας τοῖς χειρουργοῖς καλουμένοις κ.τ.λ.

held that the clause hides a reference to castration—a custom which was always an abomination to the Greek. Reinhold emends the text to οὐ τεμέω δὲ οὐδὲ μὴ ἐν ἡλικίῃ ἐόντας, "I will not castrate even persons who are not grown up," a most unhappy illustration of the art of correcting corrupt texts. The insuperable objection to this view is the clause that follows: "I will give way to such as are practitioners therein." If castration be referred to, this addition is like compounding a felony, if not something worse. The writer of *Oath* would surely have said "I will not castrate," without any qualification.

The operation-clause does not appear in the Christian form of *Oath*. May it not be assumed that it did not belong to the original form, but was afterwards added to suit the prejudices of physicians at a certain period? Quite possibly it was the ban on operations noticed by Galen[1] as existing at Rome that caused the insertion to be made in our Hippocratic text. The presence of the clause in extant manuscripts of the pagan oath means merely its presence in the common ancestor of M and V, two closely related manuscripts not of the first class. We cannot therefore feel confident that it is an ancient reading, especially when we remember that on no possible grounds could the compiler of the Christian oath have objected to it. If he did not write it, it was because his copy did not include it.

[1] May it not be likely that the mediaeval distinction between physicians and "barber" surgeons began at Rome in the Galenic period? The separation of medicine from surgery, so injurious to both, is a sign of decline, and their re-union heralded in the triumphs of the modern art of healing.

Oath is the main authority for ancient medical etiquette (εὐσχημοσύνη), the other sources being *Law*, *Physician*, *Decorum* and *Precepts*, supplemented by a few remarks in Galen.

The εὐσχήμων ought not:

(1) to give poison or suggest the giving of it;

(2) to cause abortion;

(3) to abuse his position by indulgence in vice;

(4) to tell secrets, however acquired;

(5) to advertise[1];

(6) to operate—or at least to operate for stone—a rule which arose late.

The εὐσχήμων ought:

(1) to call in a consultant when such a course was necessary, and to act as a consultant when requested to do so;

(2) to take a patient's means into account when charging a fee;

(3) to be clean, well-mannered and dignified.

It is clear from a passage in Galen[2] that it was no rule of etiquette in ancient times, though it is now, to make public all new discoveries in medicine or surgery. He tells us that some surgeons concealed the persons of their patients during operations, not for reasons of modesty, but in order to prevent the disclosure of methods which they wished to keep secret.

---

1 The ἐπίδειξις or lecture was the ancient method of advertising. See *Precepts* XII.

2 Kühn XVIII pt. II pp. 685 foll.

Ancient medical etiquette was both wide and vague. It included many things which are now considered good manners, and it also banned some things which are now dealt with by the law of the State. Poisoning, for instance, and the giving of pernicious drugs could in ancient times be practised with far less fear of detection than nowadays, so that the law had to be strengthened by other deterrents.

The comprehensive nature of ancient etiquette is well shown by the clause of *Oath* which deals with professional secrecy. Such secrecy is now limited to information acquired in the course of practice. But *Oath* forbids the publication of all information "which should not be spoken of abroad," whether acquired in actual practice or in ordinary social intercourse[1].

This width of scope should be connected with the weakness of the sanction of ancient etiquette. As I have already said, the Greek doctor was not compelled to act properly; he was merely trained to consider right behaviour "good form" (εὐσχημοσύνη). Such a sanction allows rules to be general and vague; but a strong, external coercion, with the threat of pains and penalties, like that exercised by our General Medical Council, can enforce only rules that are specific, narrow and precise. Width and vagueness would lead to injustice and tyranny.

On the whole the Greek doctor responded well to the appeal to his better feelings. He was an artist first, and a man afterwards, and he called his profession, with glorious

[1] ἄνευ θεραπείης κατὰ βίον ἀνθρώπων.

arrogance, "the art." Love of the art purified and kept pure the doctor's calling when cruder means might easily have failed. At a late period in the history of Greek medicine the writer of *Precepts* sums up this typically Greek feeling in the striking sentence:

Where love of man is, there is also love of the art[1].

The age of oaths and tests seems to be passing away. They tend to become optional, and then to disappear. But they have, nevertheless, played a great part in the history of man's moral uplifting. *Oath* must have contributed much to form a high code of medical honour, even in those ages when it was no longer a test to which the graduating physician subscribed. At the present day medical ethics and medical etiquette are based upon it. Like his Hippocratic predecessors, the modern doctor refuses to shorten life, to cause abortion, and to divulge information committed to his honour; and even though doctors no longer form a brotherhood with communistic principles, they still attend the families of their fellow-practitioners without charging a fee.

In three of our manuscripts the Hippocratic oath is found in a form purposely altered "so that a Christian may take it." Two of these copies are written in the shape of a cross, and it is perhaps not fanciful to suppose that the doctor who used this form either kissed or touched the document as he made his solemn promises. At certain points there are differences of reading; either the oath had a wide circulation and these

---

[1] *Precepts* VI ἢν γὰρ παρῇ φιλανθρωπίη, πάρεστι καὶ φιλοτεχνίη.

differences arose gradually, or else several independent forms were current at one and the same time. In either case the vitality of the oath is clearly shown.

Unfortunately, although we can date the manuscripts in which this oath appears, we cannot say when it was first composed. If, however, all our three manuscripts are descended from a common archetype, this archetype was probably written some centuries earlier than the tenth, the date of the earliest manuscript.

A minor but interesting peculiarity of the Christian oath is that it omits the operation-clause. Apart from this the chief differences between the two forms are these. The Christian oath omits:

(1) references to pagan deities[1], which obviously had to be omitted;

(2) all the clauses in which preferential treatment is promised "to my teacher, his sons, my sons, and to those who have sworn allegiance to the physicians' Law";

(3) reference to a $\mu\iota\sigma\theta\grave{o}s$ for instruction; $\mathring{\alpha}\nu\epsilon\upsilon$ $\phi\theta\acute{o}\nu o\upsilon$ is substituted for $\mathring{\alpha}\nu\epsilon\upsilon$ $\mu\iota\sigma\theta o\hat{\upsilon}$.

The Christian oath makes more definite and explicit the promise not to produce abortion.

It is obvious that the most striking difference between

---

[1] In the imprecation at the end, $\beta o\eta\theta\acute{o}s$ $\mu o\iota$ $\gamma\acute{e}\nu o\iota\tau o$ $\acute{o}$ $\theta\epsilon\acute{o}s$ seems to be the first instance of "so help me God," and the addition of $\acute{o}\delta\eta\gamma\acute{o}s$ in Bonon. is an attractive variant.

the two oaths is the omission of the clauses which encouraged the formation of an inner ring of physicians from which outsiders were carefully excluded. Two alternative explanations, and two only, seem legitimate.

(1) Many varieties of the pagan oath were in circulation during the first centuries of Christianity, and one of these omitted the clauses relating to an inner circle. It was this particular form that the framer of the Christian oath happened to be familiar with.

(2) The Christian compiler purposely omitted all clauses tending to encourage a trade union[1].

It is surely obvious that the second alternative is by far the more likely.

There are one or two conclusions to be drawn which may be considered highly probable if not certain.

(1) The compiler of the oath apparently felt quite at liberty to alter the phraseology of the original, even though by doing so he did not improve the "Christianity" of it. Herein he followed the tradition of the Hippocratic text; it was not regarded with the superstitious reverence which has tended to keep comparatively pure the text of many classical writers.

[1] Professor J. S. Reid has suggested to me that the peculiar form of the Christian oath was due to the reluctance felt by early Christians to take *any* oath. See Matthew v. 34: "Swear not at all." To my mind the insuperable objection to this view is that the Christian document is most certainly an oath (it calls itself an ὅρκος) even though the actual words "I swear by —" are omitted. Professor Reid's explanation, moreover, does not account for the total omission—about one quarter of the pagan document—of all reference to the "inner circle."

(2) The compiler used a text which did not contain the operation-clause. As this clause is found in all except one of our manuscripts of the pagan oath, and in the Arabic version of Ibn abi Usaybia, it is probable that the Christian form arose before the forms containing the operation-clause ousted those which did not contain it. In other words, the Christian form is comparatively early.

(3) The compiler thought that the clauses binding the initiated student to an "inner ring" were anti-Christian.

The most fascinating problem connected with the Christian oath is why the compiler was opposed to these clauses. I once thought that the omission was due to his objection to secret societies, which were considered contrary to the Christian religion. But it is not certain that doctors formed, or were thought to form, a secret society, nor that Christians were debarred from joining such[1]. Whether or not an objection to secret societies was one reason why the clauses were omitted, there was another reason which certainly did operate. The sentences which encourage an inner circle of practitioners show an aristocratic exclusiveness, which is in sharp contrast with the universal brotherhood of Christianity. The relief of

---

[1] It might, however, be argued that, as early Christians were themselves accused of being a disloyal secret society, they would be careful to give no colour to the charge, and so be opposed to all secret societies. Again, hostility to Mithraism might develop into dislike of all close corporations. At the present day the Roman Church bans secret brotherhoods.

pain and suffering, thought the writer, should be tied by no fetters and hindered by no trade-union rules. Christian benevolence should be universal. For this reason I am of opinion that the Christian oath was written in the early age of Christianity, before the communism of its first devotees, and the comprehensive range of Jesus' healing mission, were forgotten or neglected. All the evidence, without being conclusive, points to a date anterior to Galen.

SUMMARY

We know from Plato[1] (*a*) that physicians taught their sons medicine and (*b*) that Hippocrates taught outside pupils for a fee. If we combine this evidence with the account of Galen we shall infer that in the best period of Greek medicine there were exclusive schools which restricted their teaching to members of a clan (γένος) and to adopted outsiders. It is also probable, though not certain, that these adopted members swore an oath and signed a legal indenture.

In course of time a form of words would be evolved, not stereotyped, but admitting omissions, alterations or additions to suit the period, the school or the locality. The ethical clauses, however, seem never to have been seriously changed. Still it would be more correct to speak of the Hippocratic "oaths" than of the Hippocratic "oath."

The indenture would be a private agreement between master and apprentice. The oath defined the relations between the apprentice and the society into which he was entering, and laid down the rules of conduct to which that society expected him to conform. Some of the promises made might very well be extravagantly worded, being intended to be taken in the spirit rather than in the letter.

It is just possible that these societies were, in a limited sense, secret, and they certainly appear to have approximated very nearly to a guild or trade union.

[1] *Laws* IV 720 B and *Protagoras* 311 B.

We must clearly understand, however, that the extant evidence does not prove conclusively that the oath was ever actually administered. It is conceivable that it was a mere ideal, a counsel of perfection expressed in the form of an oath[1], just as many sepulchral epigrams in the Greek anthology are literary efforts which were never engraved on tombs. It is hard, however, to reconcile this view with the vitality of *Oath*, in particular with its modification "so that a Christian may swear it." Medical oaths, actually administered, are not unknown in modern times[2].

---

[1] Of such a nature do I take to be the "oath" found in several of our manuscripts (including Baroccian 204, Laurent. 74, 3, Vat. 2304, Mutinensis 61), and given by Kühlewein on page 74 of vol. I in the Teubner edition:

αὐτὸν ἐν ἀχράντοισι μέγαν θεὸν αἰὲν ἐόντα
[ὄμνυμι]·
οὔτε τινὰ ξείνων δηλήσομαι ἀνέρα νούσῳ
οὔτε τιν' ἐνδήμων ὀλοφώια ἔργα τελείων,
οὔτε τις ἂν δώροις με παραιβασίην ἀλεγεινὴν
ἐκτελέειν πείσειε καὶ ἀνέρι φάρμακα δοῦναι
λυγρά, τάπερ κακότητα θυμοφθόρον οἶδεν ὀπάζειν,
ἀλλ' ὁσίας μὲν χεῖρας ἐς αἰθέρα λαμπρὸν ἀείρων
καὶ κακίης ἀμόλυντον ἔχων κατὰ πάντα λογισμὸν
μήσομαι ἔρδειν κεῖνα τάπερ σόον ἀνέρα θήσει
πορσύνων πάντεσσι φίλην βιόδωρον ὑγείην.

[2] See J. R. Duval's *Serment*. The reader of this book finds it hard to believe that the Hippocratic oath was not a reality. I do not think that there is a copy of this book in Great Britain, but I hope to place a rotograph of it in the Cambridge University Library.

APPENDIX

It is interesting to compare *Oath* with the addresses to medical students which we find in the old medical books of India. I would note especially the "precepts" in *Charaka-Samhita*[1], one of which, "Thou shouldst never give out the practices of the patient's house,"[2] is obviously an injunction to keep professional secrets.

Even a better parallel is to be found in *Sushruta-Samhita*[3]. First is described the "initiation" of the disciple, after which the preceptor should address him as follows:

"Thou shalt renounce lust, anger, greed, ignorance, vanity, egotistic feelings, envy, harshness, niggardliness, falsehood, idleness, nay all acts that soil the good name of a man. In proper season thou shalt pare thy nails and clip thy hair and put on the sacred cloth, dyed brownish yellow, live the life of a truthful self-controlled anchorite, and be obedient and respectful towards thy preceptor. In sleep, in rest, or while moving about—while at meals or in study, and in all acts thou shalt be guided by my directions.... Thou shalt help with thy professional skill and knowledge, the Bráhmanas, thy elders, preceptors and friends, the indigent, the honest, the anchorites, the helpless and those who shall come to thee from a distance, or those who shall live close by, as well as thy relations and kinsmen, to the best of thy knowledge and ability, and thou shalt give them medicine without charging for it any remuneration whatever, and God will

[1] Part XVIII lesson viii pp. 546 foll. in the Calcutta translation by Avinash Chandra Kaviratna.

[2] *Op. cit.* p. 556.

[3] I quote from the English version edited by Kaviraj Kunja Lal Bhishagratna, Calcutta 1907 (vol. I).

bless thee for that. Thou shalt not treat medicinally a professional hunter, a fowler, a habitual sinner, or him who has been degraded in life; and even by so doing thou shalt acquire friends, fame, piety, wealth and all wished-for objects in life, and thy knowledge shall gain publicity."[1]

THE TEXT OF THE INJUNCTION OF HIPPOCRATES, KNOWN AS THE ORDER [OR ETIQUETTE] OF MEDICINE

"Saith Hippocrates:

'The student of Medicine should be gentle by birth, excellent by nature, young in years, of moderate stature and symmetrical limbs, of good understanding and pleasant conversation, sound in judgment when consulted, chaste and courageous, no lover of money, self-controlled when angered, not apt to lose his temper [even] under severe provocation, and not slow of understanding.

'He should be sympathetic and kind with the sick and a faithful guardian of secrets, because many patients tell us about diseases in themselves which they do not wish to be known to others. He should be patient of insults, because many mad and melancholic persons meet us with such, wherein we should bear with them, knowing that such conduct does not proceed from them but is really caused by a disease external to their proper nature.

'His hair should be cut neatly and symmetrically, and he should neither shave it nor suffer it to grow too luxuriantly. He should neither cut his finger-nails too closely, nor suffer them to overgrow the tips of his fingers. His clothes should be white, clean and soft [in texture]. He should not walk hastily, for this is a sign of levity, nor slowly, for this indicates faint-heartedness. When summoned to a patient he should

---

[1] Op. cit. pp. 18, 19.

sit down cross-legged, and question him about his condition with [becoming] gravity and deliberation, not in a distracted and agitated manner.

'In my opinion this way, fashion and order are indeed better than any other.'"

(Ibn abi Usaybia, p. 26.)

OATH OF THE FACULTY OF MEDICINE AT MONTPELLIER

(Pétrequin 1, p. 175)

In the presence of the masters of this school, of my dear fellow-students, and before the image of Hippocrates, I promise and I swear, in the name of the supreme Being, to be faithful to the laws of man and of honour in the exercise of medicine. I will give my services without fee to the needy, and I will never exact a higher fee than my work deserves. When I am admitted inside houses, my eyes shall not see what goes on there, and my tongue shall be silent about the secrets which shall be entrusted to me, and I will not abuse my position to corrupt morals or to encourage crime. Respectful and grateful towards my masters, I will give back to their children the instruction that I have received from their fathers. May men grant me their esteem if I am faithful to my promises. May I be covered with shame and despised by my fellows if I fall short.

OATH TAKEN BY GLASGOW MEDICAL STUDENTS ON GRADUATION

I do solemnly and sincerely declare, that, as a Graduate in Medicine of the University of Glasgow, I will exercise the several parts of my profession, to the best of my knowledge and abilities, for the good, safety and welfare of all persons committing themselves, or committed to my care and direction; and that I will not knowingly or intentionally do anything or administer anything to them to their hurt or prejudice, for any consideration, or from any motive whatever. And I further declare that I will keep silence as to anything I have seen or heard while visiting the sick which it would be improper to divulge.

And I make this solemn declaration in virtue of the Provisions of the Promissory Oaths Act, 1868, substituting a Declaration for Oaths in certain cases.

The old Latin Oath was in the following words:

Testor Deum omnipotentem me hoc Iusjurandum pro virili[1] servaturum. Victus rationem aegris commodam et salutarem praescripturum: nullius intercessione nec sponte noxium pharmacum cuiquam propinaturum; sed sancte et caste vitam artemque meam instituturum. In quascunque domos intravero ad aegrotantium duntaxat salutem ingressurum et ab omni injuria inferenda procul futurum. Quaecunque inter curandum videro audiverove siquidem ea efferre non expediat silentio suppressurum.

See also ARCHIV FÜR GESCHICHTE DER MEDIZIN XI p. 318 (Leipzig 1916) *Eidesform für Ärzte, Apotheker, Hebammen.*

---

[1] Should not *parte* be added?

SELECT BIBLIOGRAPHY

For notices of the less important editions see E. Littré *Oeuvres complètes d'Hippocrate* vol. IV pp. 626, 627 and J. E. Pétrequin *Chirurgie d'Hippocrate* vol. I pp. 177–180. See also the editions of Hippocratic works by F. Z. Ermerins and C. H. T. Reinhold.

1643. I. H. Meibomius. *Hippocratis Magni ὅρκος sive iusiu-randum.*

1751. Fr. Boerner. *Super locum Hippocratis in iureiurando maxime vexatum meditationes.*

1818. J. R. Duval. *Serment d'Hippocrate, précédé d'une notice sur les sermens en médecine.*

1849. Francis Adams. *The Genuine Works of Hippocrates*, vol. II, pp. 777–780.

1913. T. Meyer-Steineg, W. Schonack. *Hippokrates über Auf-gaben und Pflichten des Arztes* (Kleine Texte).

1921. C. Singer in R. W. Livingstone's *The Legacy of Greece*, pp. 213, 214.

1921. O. Körner. *Der Eid des Hippokrates.* Vortrag.

1923. W. H. S. Jones. *Hippocrates*, vol. I, pp. 291–301, and vol. II, pp. 259–261.

See also the article "Hippokrates (16)" in Pauly-Wissowa's *Real-Encyclopädie.*

Printed in the United States
By Bookmasters